Generating Joy

Release the Struggle,
Embrace the Mystery

Suzanne Schevene Brokaw

Intuitive Artist & Author
Intentional Creativity Instructor &
Guide in Holistic Living & Energy Awareness

Author Name
Suzanne Schevene Brokaw

Publisher Name
Awakening Essence

Contact Information
https://www.awakening-essence.com

Generating Joy / Suzanne Schevene Brokaw —2nd ed.
ISBN 979-8-9870219-2-7

Limits of Liability and Disclaimer of Warranty

Table of Contents

Dedication

To all those taking a stand
for deeper levels of care,
connection, creative
& well being

Introduction

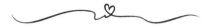

I was in the 7th grade when we had to write a paper on what we wanted in life. I was pleased with what I wrote as I handed it in, however it was returned to me to re-write simply because what I desired in my life wasn't an acceptable pursuit. I wanted to be happy.

I believe that happiness, or more precisely joy, is an innate part of living on this planet. Joy is one of those things people desire but it is often mixed up with instant gratification, momentary happiness and reaching goals. Therefore, it is often seen as a passing experience that one must continually maintain.

Happiness can come and go, but true joy is an inner state of being that can feel like delight, fulfillment, inner peace or contentment. It is rooted in a sense of connection with self: who we are, what we desire and what gives us meaning.

It isn't a passing experience. It is a way of being. It's an inner aspect of who we are and when we have the freedom to express our authentic self, we have access to our innate joy. The doorway to joy through self-expression is accessible to everyone.

A common place we get stuck, therefore unable to reach our real joy, is when we pretend to be something we are not. When we try, try, try and continue to feel less than.

And we struggle – to be good enough, to stay safe, to be worthy, to get the money to pay our rent and so on.

It isn't easy. Most of us have struggled with these things. Many of us have worked hard to pay rent, feed our children and keep our heads above water. Trauma lives, to varying degrees, in most everyone.

Struggle has often been a normal way of being.

It takes conscious effort to shift a lived experience and belief system from struggle to something better. Going from struggle to joy in one step would be delightful albeit unlikely.

It is a journey that gets brighter with each step, but it is YOUR journey and you must take those steps. However, know that you are not alone.

As we begin to embrace the mystery, we begin to steer, not control, our lives. Those who try to control their lives find their world getting smaller and smaller as there is so much effort going into controlling that there is little energy for anything else.

We are not in control of all that happens, but we are in charge of how we respond to 'all that' and what we choose to do about it. I wrote the first edition of Generating Joy thirteen years ago to guide others towards a lighter way of being in the world; one with more joy. It's time for an update.

My intention is to inspire you towards developing a more joyful life by shifting your perception from struggle to one of curiosity about the mystery of it all and beginning to engage life in a new way.

Welcome to the journey - a journey towards joy.

How to use this book

Although it builds as it goes, you may open to any section and use the inquiries in a way that suits you.

It would be helpful to have a journal to explore your thoughts and ideas as you go along through writing or even sketching. You could also use the inquiries in a walking or sitting contemplation. Let go of figuring it all out and allow your deep inner knowing to arise and be expressed.

Ask the question. Listen. Be curious.

Notice what shows up.

The point is to outwardly express what is showing up on the inside to witness, release, understand and accept or somehow interact with what your inner Self is needing to explore and express.

As always, be gentle with yourself.

A *Life by Design*

Imagine going about your life in a way that feels nourishing and nurturing. From this place of fullness, you tend to what truly matters to you, engaged in activities that light you up and allow joy to emerge.

How does that feel in your body?

The wonderful thing about this is not only do you feel empowered to express yourself, but buoyant in joy as you follow your inner guidance, building trust, resilience and resourcefulness. You are building a lifestyle that breeds joy.

Welcome to the world of Joyful Living.

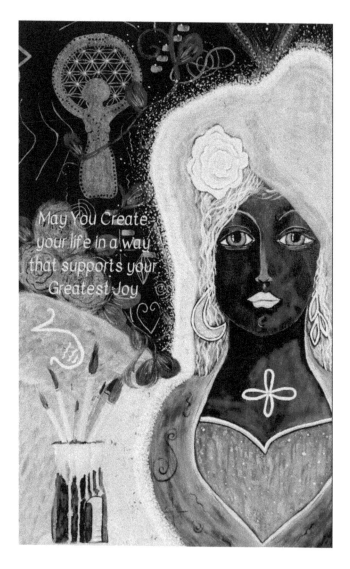

She Who holds Wisdom & Truth
What is ready to be revealed?

Awakening to Self

Journey towards Joy

What do you long for,
really, truly long for?

Do you know?

This is a question few can readily answer
initially. We are taught to look outside of
ourselves for answers and guidance. When we
are young this is important.

Yet, as we grow and explore, the path to true
sovereignty lies in learning to turn inward—to
tap into our own dreams, desires and deeper
wisdom.

But do we?

Too often we don't. We linger in the confusion, the pain, the places where we feel lost. Moving beyond these stuck places is part of the journey toward knowing ourselves—our true needs and desires, our dreams and intentions, our likes and dislikes. It's only then that we can begin to sink deeper into our unique and authentic life.

Coming home to the Self is an act of courage, a declaration of self-worth and authenticity. It's about shedding the old narratives that no longer serve us and opening to new possibilities that are waiting to be explored.

When we turn toward ourselves, we are taking a bold step—choosing to reconnect with who we are, what we want and how we intend to live our lives. On this path, we start to question the old struggle stories that, while once true for us, may no longer serve. As we choose new stories, we discover more of who we are and who we're becoming.

Be open to the possibility that your old stories, while once valid, are no longer relevant. Yet, the habits and patterns remain until we consciously turn inward with loving kindness and compassion. By seeking connection within and making new choices, we come home to our true Self—the one unshaped by others' expectations. And this homecoming leads to joy.

As we awaken to more of our authentic Self, the world grows brighter. We become curious about our unique expression and find ways to share that light with others. In doing so, we ignite joy in those around us, creating ripples that spread far beyond ourselves.

Turning toward ourselves is a bold, necessary decision. It's a way of claiming that we matter, that our needs and desires are worthy of attention, nurturing and love.

And as we claim that for ourselves, we also claim that for others. Let us be a stand for all to embrace the truth of who we are and to live the lives we desire, in peace, joy and love.

It's not what you are that holds you back,
it's what you think you are not.
-Denis Waitley

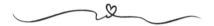

Who are you? Who are you to think that you can change? Who are you to think that you can change your world?

You are the only one that CAN change your world, for it is through your early experiences that false beliefs were created and they grew as you grew.

As the outdated beliefs, old stories and traumas are released, you are then free to experience the deeper truth of who you are and to live your life in a new way.

How does that feel in your body?

Pause. Breathe. Read it again, out loud.

Consider putting on some delicious music and dance. Feel the beat, the rhythm, the harmony, your connection to the earth, to yourself and to life.

continued ...

In this moment, know without a shadow of a doubt that you are a powerful source of creation in this world.

You are a gift unlike another, and what you express can only come through you, for you are unique and wonderful. And this gift is not only for you but for those around you.

You are the only one that CAN change your world! Is it time for a shift?

Let your heart be your compass.
Your mind you map.
Your soul your guide
& you will never get lost.
- Ritu Ghatourey

Some things cannot be discovered until we have been stuck, incapacitated, or blown off course for a while.
-David Whyte

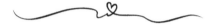

What if you gave yourself the daily gift of reflection time to reawaken your inner world?

What if this time helped you return to your path, your true north, with the wisdom you gained from being stuck or blown off course?

Imagine using that wisdom to build bridges instead of walls. What might that feel like?

Reflection time offers a break from the demands of the world. Many people find this space through meditation or journaling.

For me, walking and/or journaling helps empty my mind, organize thoughts, and explore new ideas forever flowing through my awareness.

The key is to not get caught up in the initial thoughts or distractions. Notice them and let

continued ...

them float on by, or funnel them into your journal, an audio recording or any method that works for you.

Once those things are cleared out, you can sink into the quieter places within, where deeper truths and wisdom reside. It is through listening to your intuition and responding in a fully expressive way that you discover and return to your most authentic self.

When we externalize our sense of self, we lose connection with that inner relationship. But when we turn inward and honor who we truly are, we not only offer ourselves a gift, but we share that gift with those around us.

Come back home to yourself. Feel the peace, the joy and the connection that is waiting for you. Know that you are wonderfully unique, and what you express in this world can only be expressed by you - no one else can do what you do in the way you do it.

Create Sacred Time & Space

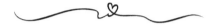

Experiment and notice what activities take you beyond your daily routines and into a realm of expansiveness and tranquility. It could be regular walks, journaling or any type of creative expression that allows you to be wholly absorbed in the process.

Painting quickly takes me out of time and space where I can absolutely enjoy myself expressing through color, marks, shapes and layers of paint. I can paint how I'm feeling. I can ask a question then let it go and usually an answer shows up. I can journey through a healing process. It is one of my favorite happy places (as long as I don't judge myself).

Regarding any new activity, it isn't about doing something well. It's about the process of exploring and expressing from within – of getting to know yourself at a deeper level.

Be gentle and allow yourself the space to explore, be curious and just see what happens.

Self honesty is a tool without which you will find it very difficult to grow. Without it, you find that you disguise and dress up the reasons for your actions and reactions in order to feel acceptable and worthy to yourself and others. By being honest with yourself you have the most wonderful tool to discover your secret fears and hidden beliefs about yourself and your reality. In the embracement of those fears you become centered and strong. This is called sovereignty. -P'taah

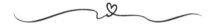

Trust in Self is vital, for if we cannot trust ourselves who can we trust? It begins with saying what you mean and meaning what you say, to yourself and others.

Be honest with yourself and trust will build. Building trust is essential for healthy nurturing relationships whether it is your relationship with yourself or with another.

Do you say you will do something, knowing full well you won't? Do you use the word 'try' as an excuse not to do it when the truth of the

continued …

situation is that your heart just isn't in it and you have no interest in doing it? How might it feel instead to say what is true –

- My heart isn't in it.
- It's not a priority for me.
- I don't have the energy for that right now.
- No thank you.

The first step is a willingness to observe yourself with curiosity. You will need to feel safe, heard, and valued for who you are. This may happen during your alone time or with the support of a healer, coach, or mentor.

Start small and be gentle with yourself. While you don't need to explain yourself to anyone, if you've been saying 'yes' all along and now you say 'no thanks' the other person may be confused. You can simply offer that you are listening to yourself more intentionally now or you are being more discerning around how you spend your time and energy or you're developing new skills and learning to say no.

continued ...

You will find that with practice your skill of self-honesty and the resulting self-trust will serve you well in all aspects of your life.

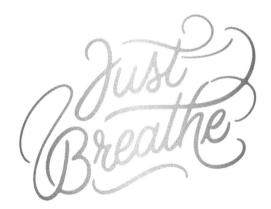

Breathe!

For Relaxed Concentration

Two facts: It is not possible to feel anxious while breathing abdominally. If you tell the truth, your body relaxes slightly. So, take a big belly-breath and after the out-breath, say something true. Anything will do but it must be unarguable.

Today is Tuesday. I'm sitting in a chair.

Keep it simple. Just take a deep, relaxed, full breath, and tell the truth. This puts the body and mind into alignment, freeing your attention to focus on the task at hand.

Chest-breathing is wired into the anxiety-producing mechanisms of the body, while belly-breathing is wired into the relaxation-producing mechanisms.

Simply by breathing deeply, into your belly, you will notice changes in your physical, mental and emotional well-being.

continued ...

When you need to Let it Go

Catch yourself as soon as possible after a negative experience, take 3 deep belly breaths, and change your body position (shake it off, stretch, jiggle - do what works for you). Part of the mechanism of a bad mood is shallow breathing and frozen body postures; don't let the negativity settle down into your body. Keep the energy moving on its way.

The human body is designed to discharge 70% of its toxins through breathing. Breathe deeply and let go.

Typically we breathe into our chest rather than our belly , resulting in a fraction of the oxygen getting into our blood system (less than 1/10 liter of blood flows through the top of the lungs – the chest breath, as opposed to over a liter through the bottom of the lungs – the belly breath) which causes the heart to work harder.

Help your heart & breathe deeply – it matters!

***The biggest communication problem is
that we don't listen to understand.
We listen to reply.***

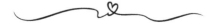

Do you really listen or do you simple hear?

I can hear what you are saying, nod my head
and wait for my turn to talk.

Or I can listen - to what you are sharing,
witness how it is for you and be present to
your message, including that which is beyond
the words. And then I can respond.

Which would you prefer?

Be the person who listens truly listens—to
understand. First to yourself, then to others
and all of life. When you do, you open the door
to profound growth and understanding.

Wholeness or health is our natural state. The nature of healing involves removing obstructions to this natural state and bringing individuals into alignment with themselves and their world. Free of these obstructions, an individual's innate intelligence and self-regulating capabilities will guide him/her toward a state of well being. – Richard Carlson, PhD

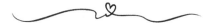

Health is often viewed as simply physical, but it encompasses much more. It is about being in harmony with life—physically, emotionally, mentally, and spiritually.

Wholeness emerges when we engage fully with life. Healing, then, is the removal of obstructions that block our natural flow.

When we release these blocks, our innate intelligence can guide us toward well-being. Healing is not about fixing what's broken but restoring the flow of energy and vitality by addressing underlying imbalances. It's about

continued ...

reconnecting with life's rhythms and finding alignment.

While full recovery from an event may not always be possible, healing can unfold regardless. Think of your well-being as a symphony of interconnected parts—immune system, nervous system, nutrition, and sense of self. Each plays its role in orchestrating wellness.

Perhaps your body needs nourishment, your mind craves stillness, or your spirit seeks connection with nature. By tuning in and responding with care, you can allow healing to happen naturally, a return to your innate state of balance.

Listen closely to your body's whispers, and with gentle attention, move toward wholeness. Trust your intuition and take loving steps forward. True healing is a journey of self-compassion, allowing your natural state of wholeness to reemerge.

Honoring Us

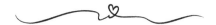

You are unique. You bring something into the world that no one else possibly can. Though we may do the same things, the results will always vary because each of us adds our own flavor of creativity and brilliance to whatever we touch.

Think of our hands. They are very similar in design yet when you look closely, they are indeed different. Similar in structure but varied in detail.

Honor your uniqueness. Honor my uniqueness.

Let's celebrate what we share and honor what differentiates us. It is through this diversity that we enrich one another and contribute to the whole.

We are unique and united at the same time—each bringing our gifts to the collective table of life.

What Size is Your Box?

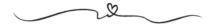

We all have limitations, whether we've created them ourselves or adopted them from others.

The key is recognizing that we have the power of choice to live within the limits we've set or to expand them.

For our children, we set boundaries to help them grow safely. As they mature, we expand these boundaries to allow them to take more responsibility for their actions.

As adults, we often build our own limitations or live within those limitations set by others.

Some "limitation boxes" are small and made of steel, others are large with perforated sides so that we can peek beyond their structure yet remain safely inside. Some have doors so we can go out and explore and have a safe place to come home to and others seemingly have no sides or walls at all and anything goes.

continued ...

We create them to make order of our world and to function within it.

The freedom comes in recognizing that we have the power to change the size and structure of our box at any time.

How do you feel about what you've created? It is time to make any adjustments?

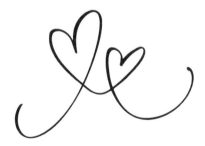

When you have freedom to fail you can
welcome the joy & freedom to succeed.

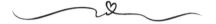

When did we accept the idea that failure is a bad thing? Have you EVER tried something new and succeeded on your first try? I sure haven't and I believe it is an expectation that hurts us in many ways. It dampens our enthusiasm to try new things, it feeds into the inner voice of not being good enough, it can move us into envy of those who are doing it well (and have "failed" many, many times) and keeps us separate from others.

But what is failure, except the perspective that we didn't meet our high expectations instantly. This is how we learn; we fall short, become curious, utilize our creativity to make the needed adjustments and try again.

And for those fellow life-learners, this is life. Our curiosity leads us to try things, our humor keeps our 'failures' light and adventuresome, our creativity spurs us on to try it again in a different way and we step into the mystery of what might be.

continued …

When we are afraid to fail, we automatically cut ourselves off from so much. Be free to fail.

How?

1. Try something new: Do something, anything (sing a song, draw, paint, cook), without any expectation of it being anything other than a fun thing to try. Let it be awful and feel the inner joy of pure expression without attachment.
2. Question the fear: Journal 'what if I fail, then what?' and when you get an answer, ask again "so, if that happens, then what?" and keep going until you get to the root cause, which is often much less dire than you might think. In most cases, failure won't hurt you, so why not try?

The reason it's important to embrace failure is that fear of failure is the number one block to trying new things and trying new things is what we need to do in order to find our voice, our freedom and our joy.

What am I feeling?
What do I need?

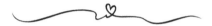

Do you know what you truly feel and need, beyond ego, addiction or habit? These are questions that go deeper, requiring you to pause and listen.

Ask more deeply. Take time to listen. Anytime throughout your day, when you awake or before you fall asleep, ask these questions.

When you react to a situation, you're often not connecting to the actual feeling. Instead, the automatic reactions—rooted in old patterns—take over (road rage is one example). You are no longer in charge. You bypass the conscious brain and react via autopilot fueled by the false beliefs created when you were young.

Or perhaps you've locked away your feelings and use distractions to endlessly distract yourself. Anything can work – food, drugs, shopping, television - there is a plethora to choose from. This too is a way of not actually feeling what is going on within yourself.

continued ...

Before reacting to someone or a situation, pause, take a few nice deep breaths and ask "What am I feeling? What do I need?" Listen, then respond with awareness.

Feelings can only evolve if they are being felt.

With practice, you'll begin to open the door to deeper layers within yourself, places that long to be acknowledged.

Ask the questions, and then begin to build bridges to a fuller, more authentic relationship with yourself.

Within you there is a stillness and a
sanctuary to which you can retreat
at any time and be yourself.
-Hermann Hesse

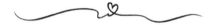

How do you reach your inner sanctuary?

You want something that takes you out of your head and your day-to-day stresses and into something more expansive.

A quiet walk in nature, meditation, body or energy work, dance, watching clouds perhaps.

Creative work also does this. You can be like a child discovering your world for the first time, totally focused on what you are involved with. It is not about what your creation looks like, it is about the process of creating.

Perhaps your creative activity is in the form of writing, painting, dancing, singing or playing in the mud – whatever it is, it must have a very large feel good factor to it.

continued ...

When you are in that space of feeling good, deeply engaged in your activity, you are not bound to the debilitating aspects of the world around you, but you are tapped directly into Source, God, whatever you call it.

A time and place to nurture your Self in a way that only you can.

Take the time. Be in your creative joy.

It matters. You matter. A lot.

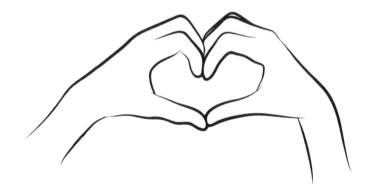

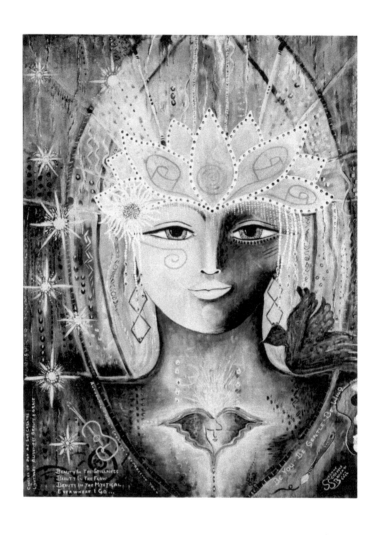

She Who holds Creative Inspiration
Is it time to listen to your one true voice?

Cultivating Inner Connections

Nurture Your Inner Sanctuary

Connect first with self, for we must connect within to weather the storms of life guiding us towards greater wholeness.

As we connect within and learn to listen to our inner world, we begin to build resilience, resourcefulness and responsibility. Our resilience allows us to bounce back while our resourcefulness helps us find what we need and, of course, our responsibility is the ability to respond.

How do we do that? By slowing down, allowing ourselves the space to just BE and notice what arises. Then listen. It may take time if this is new and that is ok.

Many are familiar with the critical voices within and less so with the supportive voices. We've fragmented ourselves over time as we have attempted to lock away those parts we or others have deemed less desirable.

We show various parts according to the roles we play (business owner, mother, friend..) and often those too are fragmented.

I am saddened when I hear people talk about wanting to get rid of parts of themselves. The ego is bad. The critical voice needs to be eliminated. And so on.

These parts are us too! We need the ego or we wouldn't bother getting out of bed. The critical voices are doing their best to keep us safe and/or to get a message to us. Do we listen? Do we ignore? Do we beat ourselves up for the fact that they exist?

The image of a devil on one shoulder and an angel on the other is something most of us have seen in cartoons or expressed in a myriad of ways. This or that? One or the other. One wins, one loses. Yet, when they work together, the best is expressed utilizing the wisdom of both.

The critical part, often seen as the devil, tries to stop us in an attempt to keep us safe. This, of course, is based on past experiences which is all it has to go on. It doesn't have the capacity to think new thoughts or understand the need for adventure.

The muse, or angel, on the other hand, is all about being in the moment and exploring new lands. The muse wants to try new things, to explore, to play, to be uplifted and inspired.

Consider cultivating self-compassion and acceptance by acknowledging that every aspect of Self is valid, has something to offer and is worthy of love.

By integrating our various inner voices we find harmony within ourselves, wise guidance and deep love.

Many today feel a sadness we cannot name.
Though we accomplish much of what we
set out to do, we sense that something is
missing in our lives and – fruitlessly –
search out there for the answers. What's
often wrong is that we're disconnected
from an authentic sense of self.
-Emily Hancock

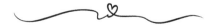

In what ways do you connect with yourself?
What feels deeply nurturing and nourishing?
What feels your soul? Where does your mind,
body and spiritual nourishment come from?

Take daily time for yourself. The importance of
slowing down and connecting within builds
essential qualities for navigating life

Take a walk in the woods or by the ocean or in
a field and reconnect with the earth.

Ground. Replenish. Restore.

Nature offers an abundance of support and has
a natural ability to bring us back into balance

continued...

and into a state of peace. From there, sense inward.

Maybe it is time to let go of the story that you are alone or not good enough or don't matter: Journal, use sound (hum, sing, scream, make the sound that you are feeling within to release it), write a "get it out" paper then burn it to release the energy.

Letting the anger, sadness or hurt settle into your body and energy field creates problems, so please, let it go.

Release can happen when you provide an avenue for the energy to flow out. Whatever is keeping you from connecting to your authentic sense of self is not serving you any longer.

It's time to release the blocks, allow the flow and connect within.

It matters. You matter. A lot.

Full to Overflowing or an Empty Barrel of Apples?

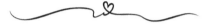

Are you able to maintain your fullness and presence with yourself and others? Or are you feeling ... you know, the other one?

As we come to realize that an empty barrel has no more apples to give, hopefully we also come to understand the real necessity for self care.

There are many ways to do this and you probably have your favorites. What is important is that you remember to keep yourself full to overflowing, so that you can offer the best that you have to give.

Here are a few reminders:

- Trusting the existence of nurturing life force energy allows you to recognize that you are loved and supported throughout your life, and allows you to live from trust rather than from fear.

continued ...

- Feel the presence of this life force energy in your body as a natural state of being to help open your awareness to the sense of belonging, reclaim your inner wisdom and experience vitality and joy.

- Integrate this energy throughout your entire system to help you establish a full personal container with strong, flexible, healthy boundaries.

- Expand your perceptual lens to see clearly, release expectations and limiting beliefs and open fully to life.

- Choose nourishing resources moment to moment to provide for yourself a steady foundation and inner peace.

Integrate ways into your daytime routines to keep yourself full. Not only will your life be that much better, but it will ripple out to others as well. And it will ripple out from them to others. And from them... And from them...

Throughout our lives, we are guided and directed by others. There comes a time when we must follow our own inner compass. By listening to your heart and following its gentle wisdom, your inner compass will guide you in the direction of your dreams. Find your 'true north' and follow where it leads. Trust that it will take you where you need to go. -P'taah

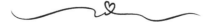

It's time to return home to yourself, find your true north and set sail anew.

- Become self aware and tend to your needs and desires. Begin by asking yourself throughout the day: How am I feeling? What do I need right now? What do I want? Or you may want to do daily journaling as you explore more of your inner world.

- Connect within and become present to what is going on. You don't need to change or fix anything at this point; just be with it. Sometimes your presence is all that is needed for a shift to occur.

continued ...

- Return to your body and integrate your awareness. Many of us have disassociated with our bodies and if that is true for you, can you now begin to bring yourself back home to your body?

- Feel the awakened potentials within you. Can you feel a deep inner urge for some unnamed something? It usually starts as a feeling and slowly comes into view. Be curious and notice what calls to you.

- Claim your dreams and set sail in that direction. Life isn't a straight line but when we know our direction, we can flex and adapt as necessary.

Receiving body or energy work can help with all of this. Sad to say, but holistic care is still seen as an oddity in this country rather than the long time valuable resource that it truly is.

And as wonderful as our medical system is, 70% of our unhealthy people have conditions

continued ...

which are outside the range of the medical community's expertise.

If need be, create your own team to help with your healing and your journey back home to your body. Too many people are unaware of what is happening from their neck down. They live in their head or out in the ethers.

It's best to be well grounded in your body as a home base and to sail forth from there.

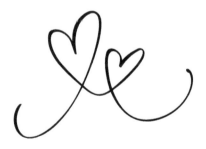

Not everything that is faced can be changed.
But nothing can be changed until
it is faced. -James Baldwin

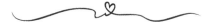

If frustration and anger are building, first off Breathe!!! Slow, deep breathing. Then try something that doesn't require quick thinking or decision making like walking or swimming.

If stress and responsibilities are building, go for something that requires concentration to give you a break, such as zumba, archery or circuit training.

If you feel vulnerable, you might consider taking on a challenging activity such as a new class, weight training or skiing to strengthen muscles, mental fortitude and improve self image.

If you feel tired and your energy levels lag, take a break and stretch, walk, dance, sing, close your eyes and focus on deep breathing ... nurture yourself as best you can in that moment.

continued ...

And in general, I find these work in every situation for me – singing, laughing, painting, being outside.

And if someone in your office stands up and belts out a few lyrics of their favorite song, just know it's all about self care. Ok, it might be a little odd, depending upon your office.

But if it DOES happen, applaud them or better yet, join them!

When Affirmations Don't Work

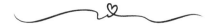

Affirmation can be a valuable tool, but they can also be a source of frustration when they seemingly don't work.

Think about it: if 80% of your being feels overwhelmed, burned out and frustrated, an affirmation band-aid of "I am full of energy and enthusiasm" isn't going to cut it.

First off, it simply isn't true and your body knows it. Secondly, if you are overwhelmed, burned out and frustrated, you need to do some serious self care.

First step is to be responsible for yourself and tend to your needs. Come home to yourself, be present and take good care of yourself.

Then ask – What is true? Perhaps it isn't true that you are full of energy and drive, but perhaps it is true that as you take better care of yourself, your energy level will improve.

continued ...

So a true statement that actually feels good in your body might be:

As I take better care of myself, my energy and enthusiasm increases.

This can align all your systems in truth and the outcomes will be better.

*Every time you are tempted to react in the
same old way, ask yourself if you want to
be a prisoner of the past or a pioneer
of the future. -Deepak Chopra*

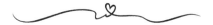

The weight of past traumas or old wounds can often act as anchors, holding us back.

We may be unable to move forward due to the heavy weights we are attached to. By releasing the energy surrounding old events that no longer serves, we can recycle that energy to be used in a more productive way.

It is at that time that the past can shift from an anchor holding us back to a source of strength, support and wisdom. Be open to receive the wisdom. Sometimes those anchors can be released out of our energetic systems without needing to relive the issue. Other times we may need to revisit and resolve something.

We all need help at times. There is no "extra credit" for a life of struggle. Why make it extra hard on yourself?

continued ...

Even with support, commitment, courage and an open curious mind is needed.

By addressing and releasing the energetic blocks, we create space for more joy and vitality in our lives.

Is it time to allow those old experiences to transform into something more valuable?

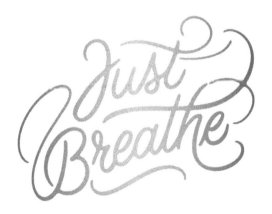

There's nothing wrong with enjoying looking at the surface of the ocean itself, except that when you finally see what goes on underwater, you realize that you've been missing the whole point of the ocean. Staying on the surface all the time is like going to the circus and staring at the outside of the tent. -Dave Berry

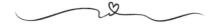

There is ample evidence (and has been for many years) about the communication network inside us. You may be aware of the power of a positive lifestyle and the impact it has on your health and overall life experiences.

Here is an exercise on how to communicate subjectively with your own body cells. This is directly from the book, The Secret Life of Your Cells, by Robert B Stone, PhD. This has been used successfully with cancer patients.

Positive belief enables your brain neurons to contact your body cells and encourage their normality. Positive mind-speak.

continued ...

Here is how, step-by-step.

1. Sit in a comfortable chair with closed eyes.

2. Relax by taking a few deep breaths.

3. Deepen your relaxation by being aware of different parts of your body—scalp, forehead, eyes—from head to toes, and relaxing these parts.

4. Imagine yourself in some peaceful place you can remember, a tranquil scene that you enjoy.

5. Pretend you are able to go into your body. In fact, you are able to be at the trouble spot in your body. Be aware of it. "See it."

6. Make corrections in your imagination. This can be as simple as seeing all cells in perfect order, working in harmony to maintain your best health—it is the concept of restoring health that is the message. Medical Practitioners call it psychoneuroimmunology.

continued ...

7. "See" any medications you might be taking working well. Love your cells and organs.

8. Imagine the trouble spot totally corrected and no longer troubled. "See" everything normal, healthy as it should be.

9. Tell yourself that when you open your eyes at the count of three, you will be wide awake feeling great.

10. Count to three, open your eyes, re-affirm you're feeling great.

I encourage you to surround yourself with positive things—people, situations, items that uplift and inspire you, all things that bring joy to your heart.

When you feel uplifted, your cells can follow suit and do their job to help keep you happy, healthy and loving life.

The 36 Jin Shin Breaths

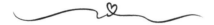

The simplest and most important self help tool we have is our breath: the inhale and the exhale.

When we exhale consciously and deeply, we release tension and stress. When we inhale naturally, we receive an abundance of life energy. This life energy connects our body, mind, and spirit.

Simply and consciously exhale while dropping your shoulders as if they were touching your feet. The smile comes naturally as you release and gently welcome the inhalation.

Each day use this formula to exhale consciously and inhale naturally 36 breaths. Full, slow inhales, letting your belly expand and feel into to the fullness. Then release out fully.

You can do this all at once or you can do 9 complete exhales and inhales 4 times per day.

Asking yourself these deeper questions opens up new ways of being in the world. It brings in a breath of fresh air. It makes life more joyful. The real trick to life is not to be in the know, but be in the mystery.
-Fred Alan Wolf, PhD

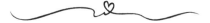

And who doesn't love a good mystery? Begin by asking the "What if" questions.

What if you knew you would succeed at anything – what would you do?

What if you really could have a life of your own choosing - what would it look like?

What if you knew beyond a shadow of a doubt that you were loved for exactly who you are right now – how would that feel?

What if you paid the bridge toll for the second car back, letting them enjoy the mystery of "who done it"? Or paid for a strangers lunch?

How might that ripple out into the world?

Forget the Words, Create the Sounds

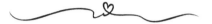

Music, sounding, vocalizing and speaking have been used for centuries to heal, calm and stimulate.

Sound literally vibrates the body. Body tissue responds differently according to the density and elasticity – muscles relax, fluids flow and nerves calm.

By producing a variety of sounds with our bodies (singing, humming, chanting, toning, sounding) we give ourselves an inner massage.

Connect with your body through sound. Find a tense area, such as the neck. Place your hand lightly on the area to focus your attention and intention. Play with sounds, pitches, rhythms until you feel the one that feels good and observe what happens.

You may find that the tension dissolves. No need to judge the quality of the sound – it's the vibration that does the job.

continued ...

Try communicating through sound only. You may want an agreeable partner for this or you will get some funny looks. Although if you growl a bit, they may immediately get it!

What is the sound of rain? Snow? A chair? Your hair? A hungry newborn? A tree? Depression? Delight? The pain in your knee?

Start using your voice in new ways and feel the freedom in your whole being.

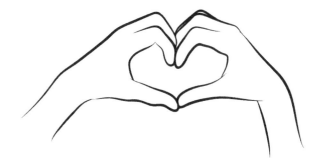

How are you? Good. You? Good.

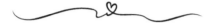

And perhaps you smile and go on your way. A co-worker of mine and I had that conversation, then we just looked at one another and laughed. It was more of a "non-conversation" than anything.

We both wanted to connect, so we both went on to share more about how we really were – our joys and challenges of what was going on.

Granted there are times when a simple greeting is all that is desired, but what if we really asked and responded with greater presence? What might that be like?

How are you?

Awesome. Everything feels like an adventure right now. I'm getting clearer on my business direction, which is inspiring to me. My body is feeling good and I feel like I'm glowing. I'm enjoy connecting at a deep level with the clients I see. Yep, life is very, very good.

continued ...

Happy? Then say so.

Why don't we share that with others when they ask? We feel it – the joy, the gratitude, the happiness inside. It wants to come out. It wants to be shared with others.

Our brain is firing smiley neurons, but our mouth is short circuiting them. Do you really want to develop THAT into a habit? Don't hide your light, your joy, your happiness.

There was a study done in Germany that stated whatever you do on a daily basis, you will be 37 times better at it in one year. That applies to even small things; it's the consistency that matters, so keep that in mind as you notice your daily habits and patterns.

If you're happy and you know it, clap your hands. Oh wait, that's song from childhood.

Well, you can still clap your hands, but also speak your truth and share your happiness.

Personal Perspectives

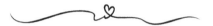

A friend of mine asked me to go SUP (stand up paddling) on the river with her; she said it would be fun.

Okay.

So as I looked around town for board shorts (in a town known worldwide for wind & water sports) all I found were clothes for size 7 and below.

A red flag went up – why is it that only small people do this sport??? Maybe there's a reason there are no larger sizes.

And I flashed back to a time when a friend of mine said to me "Hey, why don't you become a WA State Volleyball Referee with me? It'll be fun" and I'm here to tell you that being a volleyball referee is NOT what I would call fun.

All of a sudden "fun" and "personal perspective" loomed in front of me and I

continued ...

realized I didn't know what "fun" meant to Yvonne, therefore I had no idea what I was really in for. Yikes!

But out we went and as she gracefully stood up on her board and said something about it being easy, I stood up.

You know that wobble when things can either get under control or go totally out of control?

Yeah....I went out of control, bounced off the back of my board and right into the water.

I stood up, tried again (while Yvonne was doubled over laughing, still in graceful balance I might add) and with wobbly knees we paddled off into the river.

I went down again, of course, but I'm here to say that it was fun and thankfully those boards are very forgiving and supportive.

Perhaps like life.

The more pleasure I weave into my day the stronger I am. It feeds me on all levels.

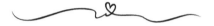

We invite pleasure in as a way to strengthen and nourish our whole Self.

It's important to distinguish between pleasure and mere leisure. While leisure activities can certainly bring enjoyment, pleasure transcends the external realm and delves into the core of our being.

It's about cultivating experiences that resonate with our essence, aligning with what brings us true joy and satisfaction.

Pleasure is not selfish or frivolous—it's a vital component of self-care and self-discovery.

By embracing pleasure as a guiding principle in our lives, we empower ourselves to cultivate a deeper sense of joy, fulfillment and inner connection.

The quality of our choices will dictate whether
we will struggle in frustration or live an
extraordinary life full of our dreams.
-Debbie Ford

While we can't always choose the events that occur in our lives, we can choose how to respond, therefore impacting our experience of the situation and the meaning we make of it.

It is the collection of our experiences and perspectives that creates our reality.

Choose wisely.
Create intentionally.
Be in the place of curiosity & receptivity.

Step back from the story, the drama, the situation. Pause. Breathe. Sense the bigger picture and the broader perspective.

When we increase our awareness, an increase in options will follow.

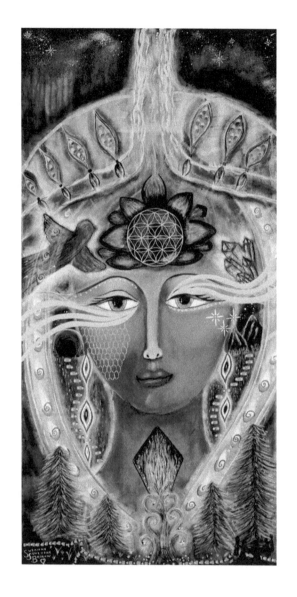

She Who holds our Wild Intuitive Self
Is it time to claim your co-creative abilities?

Discovering your Unique Brilliance

Unveil Your Authentic Self

As we begin to tap into our individuality to uncover, recover and discover more of who we are, we learn to stand in our core strength and connect with life from THAT place. And when we do that, the people, places and things we interact with are enhanced because we are more present in the current moment.

It's the journey we are on, isn't it? Many of us (including me) have been on it for decades. It's likely why you are reading this book.

But I have to tell you, I gained a whole new appreciation for the *present moment* when I acquired an ol' whack to the head a few years back. A concussion. It stopped my ability to think, forcing me into each present moment.

It was terrifying and yet, fascinating at the same time. The computer … looking down &

seeing movement as I took a step ... thinking about dinner ... all caused my head to want to explode and I'd just cry. I just couldn't handle such complex things any longer.

Fortunately I found that painting was the one thing I could do that didn't hurt my brain. That and listening to soft jazz. Neither of which I ever did before the concussion and have since learned how both calm the nervous system and enhance brain healing. Well, healing on ALL levels but my primary focus at that point was on my brain.

Painting took me to a place out of time and space, where I could painlessly create. The colors felt alive and magical. It took me to a whole new world. A world of possibilities, rich with color, full of trials and tribulations, opportunities to just be me in the moment.

After a while, I noticed that what happened on the canvas mirrored my life so well. Can I be with something that I don't like (knowing it isn't permanent) and let it be what it is? Can I allow for that? Can I let go of (paint over) something I love, to allow it to become something else, even if there isn't a guarantee that I'll like it?

Who am I in the midst of frustration when I can't express what I want to express in this moment? What happens if I simply become curious and take a risk?

When we are involved deeply with our creative expression, we enter a state of flow and it feels magical, out of our time/space continuum.

We will always reach a point that we don't like. What do we do? Throw it out? Keep going? Walk away? Who are we being in this moment of frustration, in a situation we do not like?

Can we be with something as it is, regardless of whether we like it or not? We know this is only temporary discomfort, and we aren't in any real danger.

Frustration or dissatisfaction in the creative process can serve as opportunities for growth and self-reflection. After all, it IS only paint yet the body reacts as if it matters a great deal.

This applies to any type of creative work that we love. Painting was my doorway. What is yours?

Interestingly enough, engaging in creative activities with presence and awareness can help us work through old traumas, patterns, and beliefs, leading to greater healing and self-discovery.

Accepting what is doesn't mean surrendering to it but we don't fight the reality of the moment. Right now, we don't like our painting or our writing or the way we dance. Ok. So rather than react in some way, we pause and choose how to move forward.

We may wait a day and return to it noticing what came up in our conscious awareness during that time. We may choose to continue on exploring, to learn a new skill for more satisfying results or begin to appreciate and accept something about it and come to like it as it is.

Allow breathing space. Letting go creates space for the new to arrive. Nothing in life is stagnant; everything comes and goes at some point. It just does.

Who are you in the midst of letting go? Do you tend to stand there, clutching it for dear life? Or can you appreciate what you've done and boldly step into the unknown without any guarantees of what is to come?

Any type of creativity provides a rich opportunity to learn to accept what is, to be in temporary discomfort and work within that state to change it. It's a wonderful training ground for living life in more of a flow.

Conversely, when we paint something we love and the time comes to paint over it, to let it go, can we? Are we so attached to it that we cannot bear to let it go or can we paint over it, stepping into the mystery of what is to come.

Can you let go of what you love? To be clear, you are not letting go of the love but simply the physical manifestation of it.

Can you do that and allow for the mystery?

***Sometimes it only takes a moment of
being present for trauma to release.
It's the resistance that locks it in.***

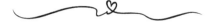

With all of these suggestions, breathe deeply
and slowly.

- Be Present. Rather than trying to get away
  from the pain, sit with it, feel it and invite it
  in to see what it has to show you. I have a
  friend who invites those uncomfortable
  parts to "come, sit, have tea and let's talk"
  to open the dialog more deeply with her
  Self. You can sit in silence or journal your
  communications. You may be surprised at
  what you learn as you open this
  connection.

- Dance with the Edges. Any kind of gentle,
  safe movement that goes to the edge of the
  pain, but doesn't force its way in can
  unlock the trauma. Yoga, slow meditative
  dance or gentle jiggles can all be effective.
  When we are fluid, it is nearly impossible
  to be pushed over. Keep the movement,

continued ...

the fluidity, go with what feels good, and allow the body to let go of what it longs to release.

- Bypass the Physical. Bypassing the physical structures and going deeper into the subtle and energetic fields and pathways create opportunities for release.

Know that trauma will release when it feels safe and when the opportunity arises. It is simply in lock down mode for one reason or another. The body will naturally choose movement over non-movement when given the chance.

Release the blocks, allow the flow, express the self.

If I continue to believe as I have always believed, I will continue to act as I have always acted. If I continue to act as I have always acted, I will continue to get what I have always gotten.

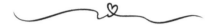

What if your story isn't true? What if it is time to broaden your perspective and see a deeper truth? Then what?

Feel the story but don't drown in it or completely believe it. Your perception is just that – your perception, but is it accurate?

Stay neutral. Open to the possibility that there are other ways to interpret the situation and allow yourself to see an expanded view.

Pause. Breathe. Ask yourself: When I open to the deeper truth beyond my initial reaction, I feel (fill in the blank).

How does that feel in your body?

Do you feel stronger, more empowered and more compassionate?

continued ...

Choose to connect to that deeper place within to create a foundation of inner peace from which to build upon.

It is through the process of listening to your intuition and responding in a fully expressive way that we discover and return to our most authentic selves. This is a gift not only for you but for those around you.

Can this be your new normal?

Don't just ask what the world needs. Ask what makes you come alive and then go and do it, because what the world needs is people who have come alive. -Howard Thurman

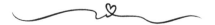

What you deeply seek is a true expression of your inner self. To express yourself is to be fully alive and the shortest route to joy.

- Claim that with is authentic about you.

- Claim your deeper truth.

- Have the courage to align with that truth.

- Be curious, be open and explore possibilities.

- Be present, generate connection and be transparent.

First with yourself, then with others and all of life. It must begin with you for unless you are at home within yourself you will always be out

continued ...

there looking for the next best thing and getting caught up in the dazzling distractions all around us.

For most, this too is a journey for we are often trained in our upbringing to look outside of self for direction, approval and reassurance that we are indeed ok.

To turn inward and ask "what do I want?" leaves many responding with "I don't know." Ok. Start there.

Begin to pay attention to yourself and how you interact with the world.

What feels good to you? What doesn't? What do you want more of and what lacks any appeal?

What makes your heart sing and allows your individual radiance to shine most brightly?

Do that. Those with open eyes will see it.

As you grow in awareness and expand your consciousness you will find that your view of your world also expands. As you view the dramas and pain and anguish of your brothers and sisters it is important that you balance detachment and compassion. It is to be in that place of support, open heartedness and unconditional love; to show forth tenderness and giving of yourself, without becoming hooked into the story; without reinforcing feelings of victimhood or powerlessness. -P'taah

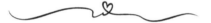

A few ways to hold your energy and not lose yourself in the story:

- Remember to breathe. You might find yourself holding your breath or holding your body in a rigid way. It's part of the fight, flight, freeze or fawn response.

- Movement always helps. Can you go for a walk and talk? If not, get some movement into your body as soon as you can. Dance. Jump. Jiggle. Don't sit in the story line and let it settle into your body.

continued ...

- Look more deeply, past the story, to see the deeper aspects of the other. Perhaps focus on their strength and courage, in spite of the situation, or any other attribute that you want to energize, helping it come to the forefront to assist them in this situation.

- Run your Core Energy, see page 106. It will help both of you to access your core centering energy more deeply.

Stand in your core strength, with the love and compassion you have to offer for a fellow traveler traversing the hills and valleys of life.

Intention & Commitment

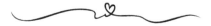

Do you make them? Do you keep them? Are you open to new twists and turns as they appear?

An intention is a direction, an aspiration, a big picture goal. It's a statement of what you are moving towards. I intend to take better care of myself or I intend to play more.

A commitment is an act of will and integrity. It is giving your word to follow through on something. I commit to working out 3 times this week or I am committed to doing something just for the fun of it every week in January.

It's important to keep your commitments - and that begins with the commitments to yourself. If you don't trust your ability to be honest and consistent with yourself, how can you trust yourself in anything you say or think, much less anyone else?

continued ...

But if there is some reason that it really can't happen, renegotiate the commitment in good faith as soon as you can.

However, committing to huge goals can be setting yourself up for failure.

Instead, intend the huge goal, but use smaller, consistent commitments to get there. One step at a time.

Just one, small committed step.

Grief, I've learned, is really just love. It's all the love you want to give, but cannot. All that unspent love gathers up in the corners of your eyes, the lump in your throat, and in that hollow part of your chest. Grief is just love with no place to go. -Jamie Anderson

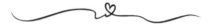

Life is full of necessary loss – the loss of a job, a loved one, an item of significance, agility or grace – it can be many things, but whenever there is a sense of loss there is a sense of grief. Something that was here is now gone.

The process of grief has many twists and turns and it is not a linear process, but there are several stages that one must travel through in order to fully embrace, release and move on from the loss.

Can we allow our feelings to be expressed, the natural process of grieving to occur and trust that the emptiness within will absolutely be filled?

Can there be space to luxuriate in the juiciness of the love we felt for what has been. Can we

continued ...

be with that? Can we allow ourselves to feel the loss without needing to replace it right now? As it releases, a heartfelt memory is gain and space is made for the next dream.

In dealing with my most recent loss, I diffused a blend of essential oils, turned on music with a strong earthy beat and cleaned house, pausing to cry as I went along. It was very nurturing and healing and exactly what I needed at that moment.

Another time I may curl up in a blanket on the couch. Different times, different needs.

The one constant in life is change. Can we honor the depth of our grief by honoring the depth of our love? Can we allow for the loss to become a heart-felt memory?

The love is still there - only the form has changed.

At some point in your life you have the choice to truly become a vibrant, whole human being.

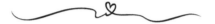

Before you reach this place, you often undergo a period of great pain, darkness or heartbreak. Few are free from this experience in their life.

In this challenge you have the opportunity to transform, which can be frightening as you move into the unknown.

It is the point where there are two distinct paths in your life. The choice is yours. Source/God/Universe holds you no matter what decision you make.

If you choose wholeness - to allow your mind to feel and your heart to think, to allow the wisdom of your history to awaken in your consciousness, to fully radiate from your core center and to step out in the fullness of who you are, you will be realizing your true potential and what, ultimately, is the answer to why you are here. Is it time to choose?

Raising our Vibration

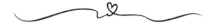

Everything in the universe is made of energy. What differentiates one form of energy from another is the speed at which it vibrates. Light vibrates at a very high frequency whereas a rock vibrates at a low frequency.

Humans vibrate at various frequencies which are determined by many factors, but primarily by our thoughts and feelings. Our primary 'home' vibration (the range we typically live in) goes out into the world and attracts energy moving at a similar frequency. Like attracts like. That's why "when it rains, it pours" and those that expect misery often get it.

And that's why raising our vibration can cause a positive shift in our life. It isn't hard to do, but it does require mindfulness.

Who is vibrant, alive and dynamic? We find them inspiring and want to be around them. And who is negative and heavy? They serve as a reminder of what we don't want to entrain to or vibrate with.

continued ...

Where do we fit into the continuum? Not as a judgment, but simply as an observation, a point of reference.

There are many ways to raise our vibration as shared in this book. One practical way is simply to consciously choose where to focus our attention.

Take 5 minutes and describe something you love love love. At the end of those 5 minutes you will feel more positive and lighter.

It doesn't have to take long to shift our energy and the more we practice it the easier and longer lasting it becomes.

Be curious.

Allow for the magic.

Allow for the possibilities.

Allow your imagination to run wild.

Begin to see the world with fresh eyes.

Thrill yourself with spontaneous action.

Allow yourself to dream the impossible dream.

Allow for the child-like wonder that is deep
within you to awaken.

Be practical. Plan for a miracle. What
could be better than that?!?

The significant problems we have cannot be solved at the same level of think we were at when we created them. -Albert Einstien

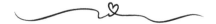

You can't have peace by fighting war—let it go and instead create peace. First within yourself, then with others and the world. But it must begin with you.

What is one action that can be taken every day that is in alignment with the more peaceful you who you are becoming?

Create peace through self awareness and connection with your inner sanctuary. As you step out into the world in your strong stance of peace and well-being, and generate connection from that place, it will be felt in a tangible way and will ripple out into the world.

Always keep your first attention on yourself. It is no longer desirable to lose oneself in another, but for each to stand in their own strength and understanding and come

continued ...

together for the mutual support of one
another.

It's time to be open to new perspectives, learn
new skills and consider new ways of being.

That is, unless you want more of the same. The
choice is yours, as always.

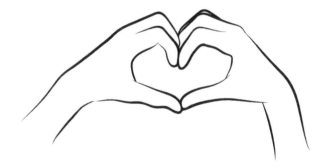

What are you beliefs about power?

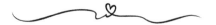

It is often used to diminish others and manipulate. Yet, true power is within and has no need to show off.

Standing in ones own power means being connected and sovereign, flexible yet strong like a tree. It's a way of being, an energy others can feel and respond to, even if no words are spoken.

We are coming into our power in new authentic ways and with more power comes more responsibility (the Ability to Respond).

Are you ready?

Our lives are inside the journey we are on. What is it like for you?

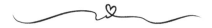

Do you need to step onto a different path – perhaps one less traveled? What would that feel like to you?

What is the story you want to live? What kind of YOU is needed for the story you are imagining for your life?

Is there excitement brewing with you? What do you stand for? What does it look like? Are you ready to take one step forward into it?

Can you reframe your journey thus far from one of victimization to one of a heroine?

Write a paragraph or two about a time when you felt victimized. Then write as much as you want, from the perspective of a heroine, about how you overcame the obstacle, developed more strength and understanding, and how you feel now. Celebrate who you are!

Mastery is the state of integration of the self. Being in one's mastery will include those triggered moments but when we are in our mastery, we stop identifying with the experience. The difference is in the perspective and way we handle it, how we embody our accountability. When we are observing, we feel the freedom to explore the experience because it becomes less serious. -Tehya Sky

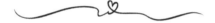

We can then embrace our imperfections with compassion and acceptance. We acknowledge our experiences reflecting our inner beauty or perhaps pointing us towards areas for growth and awareness.

As we become more present and accountable for our experiences, the need for rigid definitions of mastery diminishes.

Instead, we undergo a process of integration, gradually embodying our true selves.

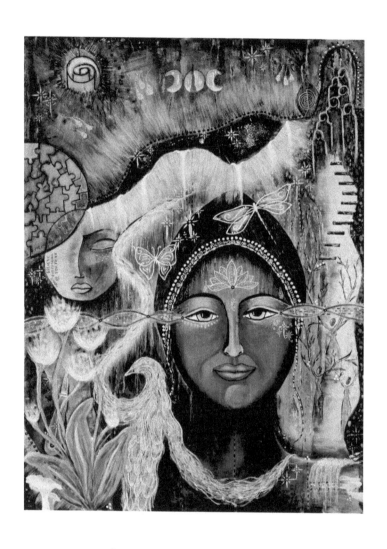

She Who holds Our Freedom
See the potential, embrace the uncertainty
& operate as the creative force you are.

Embracing your Authentic Self

Radiate Joy Within

⟋◡⟍

Standing in your core strength with the wisdom of your experiences, skills and talents is a powerful place to create from.

Take a stand to be yourself and share your unique gifts with the world! It is in this place that joy becomes a way of being that you naturally generate.

I would like to say this is quick and easy but it isn't. Often we need to unlearn and let go of what has held us hostage, be it old belief patterns, ongoing fear or negativity, lack of support ... many things can get in the way.

What perils lie around the next corner? What miracles show up when we least expect them?

The highs, the lows, the challenges, the smooth times ... this is the richness of living.

We can't always choose what happens, but we can choose how we respond and that shapes our experience, our journey.

What is calling you forth? It may simply be an undefined longing for something ... you're not sure what .. but something is stirring, something is shifting, something is happening. Can you feel it?

You don't need to know what it is .... this is embracing the mystery.

Can you simply be curious and notice? Move towards those things that appear more interesting and away from things you only do because of habit but lack any real interest. How do you choose to use your precious resource, your energy?

Explore desires, passions, longing, even if undefined at first. Choose 1 thing and explore. Cultivate curiosity and openness, guided by intuition and inner wisdom rather than concrete answers. This can be challenging when you're accustomed to thinking your way through things and reaching the 'right' answer.

How do you allocate your energy and resources aligning actions with values and passions and making conscious choices that support growth and fulfillment?

- Take inspired action towards what truly resonates with you, even if uncertain.

- Trust your inner guidance and allow Self to step into new opportunities and experiences, saying YES to life.

- Embrace authenticity and share your gifts with the world as a powerful act of self expression and self love.

- Celebrate your progress and growth along the way, acknowledging the courage it takes to step into your true Self.

When you do that, joy can follow.

And the time came when the risk to remain tight in a bud was more painful than the risk it took to blossom. -Anaïs Nin

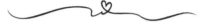

You aren't so much yearning to accomplish goals, as you are to blossom and thrive like a rose – you deeply want to bloom into the fullness of who you are, yes?

How does that feel? Does that feel true?

But like the rose bud, there are things you need in order to develop. What kinds of nourishment do you need to grow and flourish into the rich beautiful being you are intended to be?

Do you need a support system to help you stay on track? A business coach, a mentor, a holistic healer? Better self care? Time to explore your desires?

What is one step you can commit to at this time?

Walking through the Door of Change

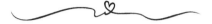

Imagine a door in front of you. It's big and solid and you have no idea what is on the other side. But it is YOUR door, and you ARE going through it.

How do you feel? Excited? Frozen in fear?

Humans resist change primarily due to fear – the fear of the unknown.

Way back in 1999, the UN's World Health organization warned of a global epidemic of depression largely due to the stress of rapid change.

Change in inevitable.

We have an evolutionary lifestyle and in order to not only survive, but thrive, we need to learn to deal with the rapid rate of change.

It isn't going to go away, nor can we succeed by trying harder to stop the changes. Our

continued ...

world will simply get smaller and our stress levels will continue to rise causing more problems – it's a vicious cycle.

How can we deal with the stress of change?

- It may mean learning new stress-reduction skills.

- It may mean learning to stay in the moment, away from fear based scenarios and limiting the influx of information.

- It may mean learning how to take risks, once small step at a time.

All of life changes, including us. Our piece is how we choose to handle it.

Are you willing to step beyond your comfort zone?

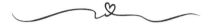

It's natural to feel discomfort or even fear, for you are venturing into the unknown, moving away from what has felt secure – a life you've built based on beliefs that may have served you well.

But now, it's time to let go of some of what has been, to make room for the possibilities that await.

What kind of possibilities? That's entirely up to you. What would feel deliciously divine?

Pause for a moment to feel, sense, or imagine that reality. You've arrived at this point through every experience of your past, each one guiding you here, to this moment. Right now.

What if you switch things up and think with your heart, feel with your mind? What if you allow the wisdom of both to work together, in

continued ...

harmony? It might take practice, but creating internal coherence can lead to profound clarity.

Now, consider: What if you let go of the struggle and instead partnered with your well-being? What if you opened yourself to the mystery of life? What possibilities would emerge? It is through exploration that you'll find them.

When you embrace child-like curiosity, when all of life becomes a miracle once more, anything is possible. Imagine feeding into the "what if" of yes, rather than the "what if" of fear. Be mindful, yes, but allow yourself to nourish the desires of your heart, those things you want to manifest.

What if we all created our lives from a place of wonder and possibility? How would it feel to create with love and innocence, just like a child? What if you trusted life to fully support you, knowing that you are connected to it all?

continued ...

How might that change the way you use your time, attention and energy?

For in your creations, life expresses itself through you, and no one else can bring forth what is uniquely yours to share.

Explore the possibilities and listen to what longs to be created through you.

What do you truly want to experience and contribute to this world?

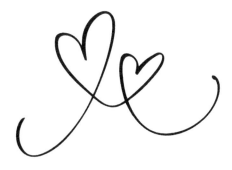

*Nature has seasons of rest and stillness,
renewal and growth. Why is it that
we think it doesn't apply to us?*

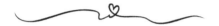

When you ride the waves you know the tides.
When you flow with life you know the seasons.

Listen and feel your way into it. You know of
this cycle but perhaps you have not paused to
remember.

All of life has a flow, a rhythm, a cycle to
maintain its harmony.

Spring brings new beginnings, new
experiences, new relationships and new
perspectives. Life is sprouting and there is
birth and creativity which is infused with
power, inspiration and energy to fuel your
passions.

Things blossom into full expression in
Summer. You are energized and motivated.
This is the force that enables your planted
seeds to grow, ripen and flourish.

continued ...

Late Summer is a time of reflection and insight. It is time to pave the way to a peaceful heart and to embrace deep gratitude for the many blessings that have come your way.

Autumn brings us to an acceptance of what is as the old is released and completed, making way for something new to be born next spring. Feel love for what has been, knowing that it is now a part of you.

Winter brings rest and hibernation. There is an awareness of wholeness, satisfaction and abundance. Peace and trust in the goodness of Life offers restoration and rejuvenation.

What season are you in right now? Immerse yourself and receive the nourishment that is offered.

Laughter...that is the great aligner! As you allow the joy and the laughter to bubble forth, there is no judgment, no fear, no limited beliefs. In those moments of great laughter you are truly in the Now, without past and without future, simply in the eternal Now in joy and alignment with your universe. In that moment your brain releases the healing chemicals which allow your body to reflect this unity in the manner of health and well-being. -P'taah

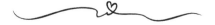

Fully live each day and be open to new possibilities that are beyond your imagination. Feel the connections with all of life and the beauty that exists all around you.

Lovingly appreciate the wonder of everything and the joy it brings. See through the eyes of a child and radiate your love outward from the core of your being.

Laugh, enjoy and find the humor in life. Be silly – be spontaneous! Feel and explore your curiosity for the wonderful, magical world you live in.

continued ...

Create for yourself a delightful morning ritual to begin the beautiful day you are about to embark on.

And perhaps an evening ritual to pause and give thanks for the blessings of the day.

Sometimes I break my days into blocks of time labeled

- Creative Expressions (writing, art, baking)
- Inspiring Actions (project work time)
- Side Quests (tasks – side quests just makes it sound more fun)
- Peaceful Pauses (reading, meditation, reflective writing).

How would you like to structure your day?

Living the Juicy Experience

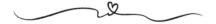

I absolutely adore the journey of personal growth and evolution. It offers me an opportunity to really love and appreciate the juiciness of healthy relationships (both with myself and others).

It reminds me of muscle tissue. Having tight, hard muscles is not healthy; there's no fluidity, flexibility, grace or ease (same with relationships).

When faced with a tense muscle many practitioners engage it head on for a battle of wits and strength to force that muscle to give up and give in. Someone wins, someone loses (muscle vs practitioner or person vs person). That's one way.

Another way, my favorite, is to graciously say hello, back off, and slide right past that tight muscle into the depths of the system to gently release from the inside out (what is the REAL

continued ...

issue), supporting the system (client or current drama) to release on its own, rather than by force, which opens the door to create a deeper, longer lasting change (into healthy muscle tissue or win-win encounter) as the new way of being ripples out to the denser structures of the body.

Perhaps that is what 'engaging with life' all is about.

Letting go of the fight, the struggle, the hardness that we've come to accept as normal and embrace the deeper feelings, the softness, the grace and ease of gentleness and begin to source our true power from there.

As Han Suyin said "There is nothing stronger in the world than gentleness."

Radiating Core Energy

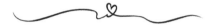

In moments when the chaos of the world overwhelms you, this tool offers a pathway to recenter and reconnect with your inner strength.

As you stand in your core strength, you also help others stand in theirs. This is easy to use in everyday situations and can be done very quickly, once learned.

Try this:

1. Grounding: Begin by directing your energy downward, visualizing it flowing out through your feet and into the earth. Set the intention for a strong connection with the center below. Take a moment to feel the stability and support of this grounding.

2. Connecting with Higher Energies: Next, direct your energy upward and out through the top of your head. Intend for a strong connection with your center above, opening yourself to the higher energies.

continued ...

Allow yourself to bask in this connection, embracing the expansiveness it brings. Allow the energy to flow through the core of your being.

3. Radiating Core Energy: Finally, radiate your core energy in all directions, envisioning it as a brilliant beacon of light. Feel the warmth and strength of this energy emanating from within you, illuminating your surroundings with peacefulness and positivity.

As you practice this exercise, you'll find that it becomes second nature to - center below, center above, and radiate core energy - empowering you to navigate life's challenges with resilience and grace.

Why Holding your Core Energy
is Beneficial for All

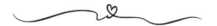

The gift in doing this multifaceted. Not only does it strengthen your personal energy field, but it supports others to strengthen theirs. Rather than putting up a shield to protect yourself from another, learn to hold your energy in a strong, solid way.

In this way you aren't building a wall around yourself. You are holding the energy and creating the possibility for another to step into a higher expression of who they are. You are building bridges instead of walls.

Imagine two people in a discussion where there is some level of disagreement. One path their discussion could take is one of escalation; each person is doing their best to make their own point which could mean their voices begin to rise, they begin to stand up taller to puff up and the defensive actions begin. Anger, frustration and righteousness may build.

continued ...

Another option is for one person to dominate the other - a classic power trip. Too often our interactions are based on some form of attempt to gain power or energy, from another. But it doesn't have to be that way.

Here's another scenario: One is standing in their power, holding strong and steady and simply listening to what the other has to say. The second person is communicating some disagreement. As the first person holds their energy without defensiveness and with a desire to understand, the second person has the opportunity to say what they need to say. They can then step up to a more mutually respectful way to deal with the interaction because the first person is holding the energy for them, helping them to move beyond the power struggle.

In this way, the relationship can progress to a deeper level of authentic communication where a win-win result is possible, with both parties feeling better as a result of the conversation.

Jewels, Jewels Everywhere

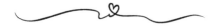

We all have them. We all share them. What's yours?

When you go into your favorite coffee shop or juice bar do you have a favorite creator of yummy drinks that you hope will be available to make your item?

Have you noticed that even though two people can use the exact same ingredients, the results are noticeably different?

What is it that really happens when you take that cup of coffee from your favorite barista? Certainly there is more than the coffee, water and cream that you receive.

There is an aspect of that barista, their jewel or energy signature or home vibration, that is unique to them and you are responding to that. It's a quality, a vibration, that you are responding to and receiving.

continued ...

How do you feel as you receive your drink? What attributes come to mind after that interaction? It could be anything - gentleness, joy, connection, integrity, lightness, humility ...

What is your jewel? What is it that people receive when they interact with you?

It is that trait or attribute that draws others to you? What is yours?

And then, how brightly do you let your jewel shine? The world needs you to shine brightly.

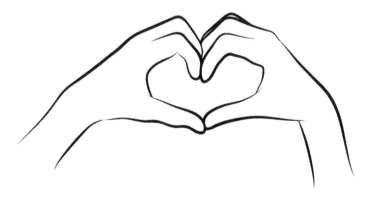

Becoming Radiant

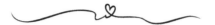

Consider Radiance—an authentic expression of who you truly are, shining out into the world, emanating from your deeper center. It's a creative energy of life that magnetizes everything and touches others on a deep, deep level. Radiance is a life force to be experienced and felt, well beyond your physical beauty.

What do you offer?

A smile? A Kind word?

An artistic design or creation?

A warm touch? A peaceful home?

Let your radiance imbue your life and

Let the entire world feel your divine radiant presence.

Vision without action is merely a dream.
Action without vision just passes the
time. Vision with action can change
the world. -Joel A. Barker

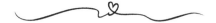

When you stake your claim in what you stand for and begin to steer your life towards your north star, your life will change. It has to.

As you claim responsibility for your actions, thoughts and false beliefs, your life will change. It has to.

As you question old habits, behaviors, interpretations of events and become curious as to what the deeper truth may be, your life will change. It has to.

As you become present with what is, reconnect with yourself and become more transparent, your life will change. It has to.

Is it time for a change?

We are living in a time of great change, personally and collectively. This time of transformation presents us with a golden opportunity to evolve beyond our current limits. If we keep doing the things we have always done, we will continue to create the same results. Do you choose to embrace your evolutionary process, or do you choose to remain the same? -Peggy Phoenix Dubro

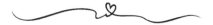

Life is an adventure and you are in charge of the trip.

Where are you now? Where are you going?

Are you planting the seeds of intention for the journey ahead into the unknown territories of possibilities? Or do you feel lost in the valley of dread?

The linear brain accesses the past to protect you in the future. So you're looking at the future through the framework of your past.

continued ...

The only time it will reach into the future to another potential is through your conscious decision to do so or some experience that pushes you there (often tragic) or through a mystical moment of some sort.

Do you want more of what has been or is it time to uplevel, ignite your life and generate your joy?

Choosing Your Path -
Embrace Possibility & Shape Reality

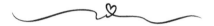

What do you truly wish to experience in life? To create? To express and contribute?

Allow yourself to consider the freedom to live fully and authentically. We say YES to our noblest behaviors because we want to, not because we have to.

As healers, bodyworkers, or simply as humans, we know the power of touch, intention, and presence. A simple gesture—a smile, a kind word, or a compassionate glance—can shift energy and transform someone's day. We all have this power, not just those of us in the field.

Will you choose to embrace this responsibility, this power to uplift? Will you embody the change you wish to see?

It starts with you. Be fully present and engage with life through intentional actions.

continued ...

In this new reality, we aren't passive bystanders. As Amit Goswami reminds us, quantum physics teaches that we are co-creators of our experience.

The choices we make and the meanings we assign shape the reality we live. It's not just about survival; it's about stepping into our power as creators of joy, purpose, and transformation.

So how will you shape your reality today?

Right now, in this moment, you get to choose. Will you choose to thrive, to embrace the gifts of life with grace and joy?

If you're feeling stuck, pause for a moment. Reflect on what truly lights you up: I love... I collect... I am inspired by... I am grateful for...

Let's make the choice to thrive, together.

Love What You Do

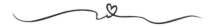

When you make what you make with love and hold the awareness that you are doing just that – creating with love - it alters the approach you take to making it as well as the outcome.

Energy is infused into all that we do, so ideally make what you make with love or don't do it (perhaps another time would be better). It does matter.

This is true for any crafted item – it carries the energy of the creator. I've had this reflected back to me regarding items I've made, even when the person noticing the energy within the item didn't know me. They still felt it.

I've recently taken on learning about sourdough baking. The Starter needs to be nourished. It needs time to integrate, grow and expand. To become what or who it is (the majority of people name their starter since it is

continued ...

much like having a child). If you don't tend to it, it will die. With love & nourishment, it will flourish.

All with the starting point of doing it with love.

May love be at the center of all choices (I put this statement on the 'Yes, I will' painting I gave to Kevin when he asked me to marry him).

Do it with love and a happy heart, knowing that you are contributing to the good vibes of all.

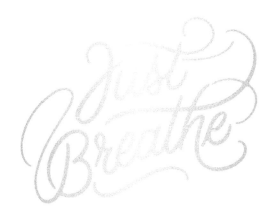

Wisdom of the North

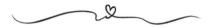

In the serene, untouched landscapes of Norway and Finland, where the air is fresh and the forests carry the wisdom of the ancients, a deep connection to nature infuses everyday life. Rooted in reverence for the natural world, the Nordic way celebrates simplicity and presence, inviting us to rediscover the beauty of slowing down and savoring life as it unfolds.

Wandering through the the lands, we are reminded of our place within the greater whole. In these tranquil spaces, we pause, breath deeply, and allow the beauty of the moment to settle into our bones.

This philosophy encourages us to embrace friluftsliv—the joy of open-air living—and sisu—the quiet, unyielding strength that lies within. It teaches us that true fulfillment isn't found in the relentless chase of achievement but in the mindful, meaningful connection we cultivate with each day. Here, productivity becomes more than just crossing off tasks; it's about

continued ...

being present, fully engaged with the flow of life and the energy around us.

These guiding principles encourage us to find balance in our pursuits, to seek fulfillment in the simple pleasures of life, and to cultivate a sense of inner resilience in the face of challenges.

Through the Danish concept of hygge, we create spaces that nurture us, welcoming stillness, connection, and warmth into our homes and hearts.

By aligning ourselves with nature's rhythms, we remember that we, too, are part of these cycles of rest and renewal. Like the turning of seasons, we honor our own phases of growth, allowing ourselves to ebb and flow with ease.

In weaving these Nordic practices into our lives—slowing down, savoring simplicity, and embracing presence—we embark on a journey back to ourselves.

continued ...

With each step we take in nature's embrace, we reclaim our connection to the earth and to ourselves, finding solace, inspiration, and joy in the beauty of the world around us.

May you BE the beauty that exists all around and within you.

The Invitation

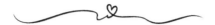

As you awaken to more of your authentic self, you begin to engage from a place of fullness and generosity. Life then becomes more graceful with a flow to it that makes even the challenges easier to navigate.

It is my hope that you learn to live within a healthy flow of energy, aligned with the truth of who you are, in service to what matters most.

We are people who want to create deeper levels of care, connection, creativity, and well being knowing that as we step into deeper authenticity, we support others to do the same.

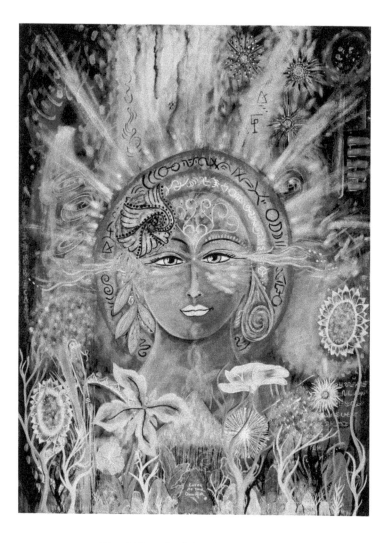

She Who holds Our Visions

Can you follow your impulses & curiosities?

Oh darling, such a rich life we live

No one likes the depths we must go
To set ourselves free, learning to flow
But in the deep darkness the power lies
To stand up, shine bright and open your eyes

Circle the spiral on your way up
To get to the answers you think are on top
But as you find Self, you will see it's not true
for all the answers lie inside of you
Lifetimes are many, wisdom runs deep
You are far more than you really think.

It is true is you are a bright light on earth
To share your fine gifts and all that you birth.
Dance in the darkness, dance in the light
Stand in your power but give up the fight
Embrace all that you are, the pieces and bits
Scoop them all in, I promise they'll fit.

Final Words

I see a world of awake and aware humans contributing to a lighter and brighter world for all. And because I can visualize it with intention, I can impact the reality of it. I can create it for myself, and then allow it to radiate out, thereby affecting a positive change in the world.

May we each BE the blessing,

Suzanne

Acknowledgment

It takes a village. How can I possibly list and thank everyone who has impacted me, all contributing to who I am in this moment?

Know that I am in deep appreciation for all of you with whom I've had the pleasure of interacting with, learning from or with, teaching to or with, or bumping into along the journey. You are a gift to me. Thank you from the depth of my soul.

About Suzanne

Suzanne has been in the health and wellness field since the early 90s as a Practitioner and Instructor. Her passion is helping others foster greater awareness, empowerment and optimal well-being in the wholeness of who they are.

She is known for her gentle presence and quiet approach to joyful living. When she isn't working on a beloved project you will find her exploring the power of intentional creativity through writing, painting, music, or cooking, enjoying the surrounding nature, inching towards slow living, or laughing at some silliness.

To see what she is serving up, please visit www.awakening-essence.com.

Suzanne Schevene Brokaw
Intuitive Artist & Author
Intentional Creativity Instructor &
Guide in Holistic Living & Energy Awareness

Printed in the USA
CPSIA information can be obtained
at www.ICGtesting.com
CBHW040918251124
17874CB00014B/174